SEEDS

from My Patients

Sasha Vukelja, M.D.

Seeds from My Patients
Published in the United States of America

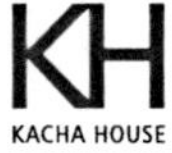

Produced with the assistance of Fluency Organization, Inc. in Tyler, Texas.
Design by Diane Kronmeyer. Cover photo: Angela Klein/courtesy of TylerPaper.com's Spotted!

This book is for you.

Live. Live! Don't just exist.

Author proceeds from *Seeds from My Patients* go to support breast cancer and cancer research.

Also available nationwide in bookstores
and amazon.com:

SEEDS: A Memoir
by Sasha Vukelja, M.D.

iPad kindle nook Reader

Table of Contents

About the Author i

Courage.. 1

Faith 13

Kindness 23

Prayer..33

Giving..43

Patience 53

Hope..63

Joy...75

Endurance...85

Love 101

About the Author

Sasha Vukelja is known to her patients simply as "Dr. V." The V stands for "Victory," a reference to her determination to fight for her patients who are diagnosed with cancer. She began writing her first book, *SEEDS: A Memoir*, over 20 years ago after the sudden death of her mother. She paints an honest portrait of a mother/daughter bond that is both poignant and painful in a book about potential and its unexpected bloom in the most unlikely of places.

SEEDS: A Memoir is the true story of how Sasha and her mother, under the watchful eye of Communists, escaped from Yugoslavia to a new life in America. In this incredible account, mother and daughter walk out of a Yugoslav prison and into the open arms of strangers across Europe who sheltered them for years at a time. They finally arrived in America with only a few suitcases of clothes, her mother's rolled-up paintings and a handful of English words. Living in a roach-infested Manhattan hotel—without jobs, family or friends—the refugees realized their fight for survival had only just begun.

In America, Sasha quietly pursued her childhood dream of becoming a physician. But she had to overcome poverty, language barriers and discrimination on her unlikely journey to becoming an oncologist.

SEEDS from My Patients is her second book and shares the priceless seeds of faith, hope and courage that her patients have planted in her life. It is a collection of inspiring stories about the power of hope, the importance of laughter and the triumph of the human spirit over difficulty. She and her husband, Dr. Larry Anderson, have two children: Maxi and Boris. They reside in Tyler, Texas.

Thank you to all of the patients and families who gave me permission to share their stories. Thank you also for endorsing the spirit of the book and seeing it as a chance for you or your loved one to inspire others who are facing the biggest fight of their lives.

I intentionally left out the names because each story is in many ways everyone's story. Some of the stories are of a single patient, but each chapter symbolizes hundreds of patients who also share similar qualities. My hope is for them to see themselves represented throughout the book as symbols of hope, triumph and courage. All of my patients are special to me, and I am thankful for the many seeds each one has planted in my life during 28 years of medical practice.

This is your story. This is our story.

Courage

Q. When should girls learn about breast cancer?

A. When they start developing breasts.

That's the message I want to get out to everyone, everywhere. Fortunately, I am not alone. My patients are some of the best educators I know.

One in particular has spread enough seeds of encouragement and hope to cover our local community and beyond. She helps educate women of every age every week about breast cancer awareness. After all, she is a teacher. And now she is a teacher with a little something extra—the extra is the courage she had inside all along. Cancer just helped her discover it.

Her story began in the most unusual way.

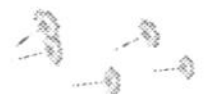

She was helping host the first-ever campus health fair for our public school district. Local health care providers were offering a number of free tests for teachers, including mammograms. Some of her co-workers were reluctant to undergo the screenings because they were on campus and not in a hospital setting. So she decided to lead by example and said, "Just follow me," as she scribbled her name beside several tests. As if it were the Olympic trials and not a health fair, she joked that she would beat them at every "event."

After she and a co-worker had their mammograms, the technician filed the X-ray films in a little black box. (On their way to the next test, she told me they guessed it would be easy to tell the films apart since her co-worker's breasts were "bigger" than hers!) They had a good laugh.

The next morning, her doctor called and said he needed to see her right away. She was not worried because she was a health teacher and had always practiced consistent exercise and excellent eating habits. But things were about to turn serious.

When her doctor walked into the exam room holding her chart, he said, "I don't have any good news for you. You have breast cancer." She was in shock. *Could it be a mistake? Did they need more tests just to make sure?* She was not ready to face reality. Things moved very quickly, and she talked with a surgeon that afternoon.

The next morning, instead of pulling into her high school parking lot for the second day of school, she was undergoing surgery. It was just three days since her first mammogram. Three days ago, she had felt healthy and strong.

The day after her surgery, the nurse came in her room to remove the bandages from her chest. She glanced down, not having a clear idea of what she was going to see. When she looked at her chest, that's when she knew what a mastectomy was. No one she knew had ever lost their breast. If they did, they didn't talk about it. It was the 1990s, and breast cancer was rarely part of public or private conversations then.

For a long time, she thought, "*This could not be happening to me. I've done all the right things. I ate right, I exercised, I've lost weight—and I've done those things for many years. Cancer snuck up on me, and there was no one I could talk to about it.*"

They told her she would need to get weighed for a breast prosthesis. She recalls thinking, *"How were they going to do that? Weigh my other breast and get me a little one just like it?"* When they told her that her hair would fall out when she began chemotherapy treatment, she wondered, *"What else would I lose?"*

When she did lose her hair, it all came out in the shower. She stood helpless and dazed in six inches of drain-clogged water trying to wipe off the clumps of hair clinging to her skin. No one she knew had lost her hair that way. It was terrifying and foreign, this fear of the unknown. As a teacher, her instinct was to open a textbook and look for answers. But this time there was no textbook. There may have been literature out there, but she did not know how to access it.

She spent almost a month recovering at home. She'd always heard that if you got cancer, you will die. She spent those first weeks doing the only thing she thought she could do: plan her death.

But she didn't die.

She lived.

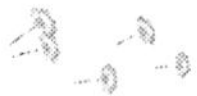

I mean she *really* began living—as if for the first time. She summoned all her courage to live for the benefit of others and to speak to them from her experience.

Together, she and I began educating women all over our community about breast cancer. They were not coming to us until they already had cancer—so we decided to go to them. We were like traveling salesmen going door to door in churches, homes and small group meetings. We carried some pamphlets and plastic breast models to show women what a lump felt like so they would know what to look for during their own breast exams. Finding the lump on the model made them more confident that they could do so at home. A lump is so often called a "silent killer" because unless you feel it, you would not know you have one.

We spread the seeds as best we could, but the lack of information (or misinformation) was astonishing. One lady told us she thought that when you received chemotherapy the doctors strapped you down on a table and injected you like an execution.

Women and men were living in tremendous and unnecessary fear of the unknown. Other women showed us their homemade breast prostheses. Many stuffed half a box of tissues in their empty bra cup or used old panties rolled up in a bowl or a wad of sanitary napkins. Another woman at a meeting raised her hand to ask a question and birdseed spilled out of a baggie she had used to form her missing breast. My patient graciously removed her silicone breast prosthesis from her bra, laid it on the table beside her and let other women examine it. It helped them understand there were much better alternative breast forms than birdseed and tissues. Some timidly asked to see her mastectomy scar, and she willingly showed them so she could educate them.

We also traveled together to several Susan G. Komen Race for the Cure events that were raising breast cancer awareness in other big cities nearby. I remember piling into her van with several other cancer survivors to run the race and talk with organizers about how we could bring Race for the Cure to our city, too. In 1999, after more than a yearlong application process, Tyler hosted its first Race for the Cure and over 2000 people participated. We hugged and cried when we saw all the pink shirts streaming into the street that day for a common cause.

It's one thing when a doctor talks about breast cancer—it's entirely different when another woman speaks from her own experience. "I'm not a doctor. I'm another woman," she often says. "Our cancers may be different. Our recoveries may be different. But we're the same in a lot of ways." People who are battling cancer have to dig deep just to find enough courage to get themselves through it. It's really extraordinary when they dig deeper still and start to fight for others. That's the next step. As a teacher, she just considers the community a larger classroom. She gives out her phone number at small groups and meetings and tells patients to call her 24 hours a day if they need to talk. Cancer is not who she is—but she doesn't want to forget it. It changed who she was. For the better. She was always a good teacher. But now she is a *great* teacher.

Always seek out the seed of triumph in every adversity.
—Og Mandino

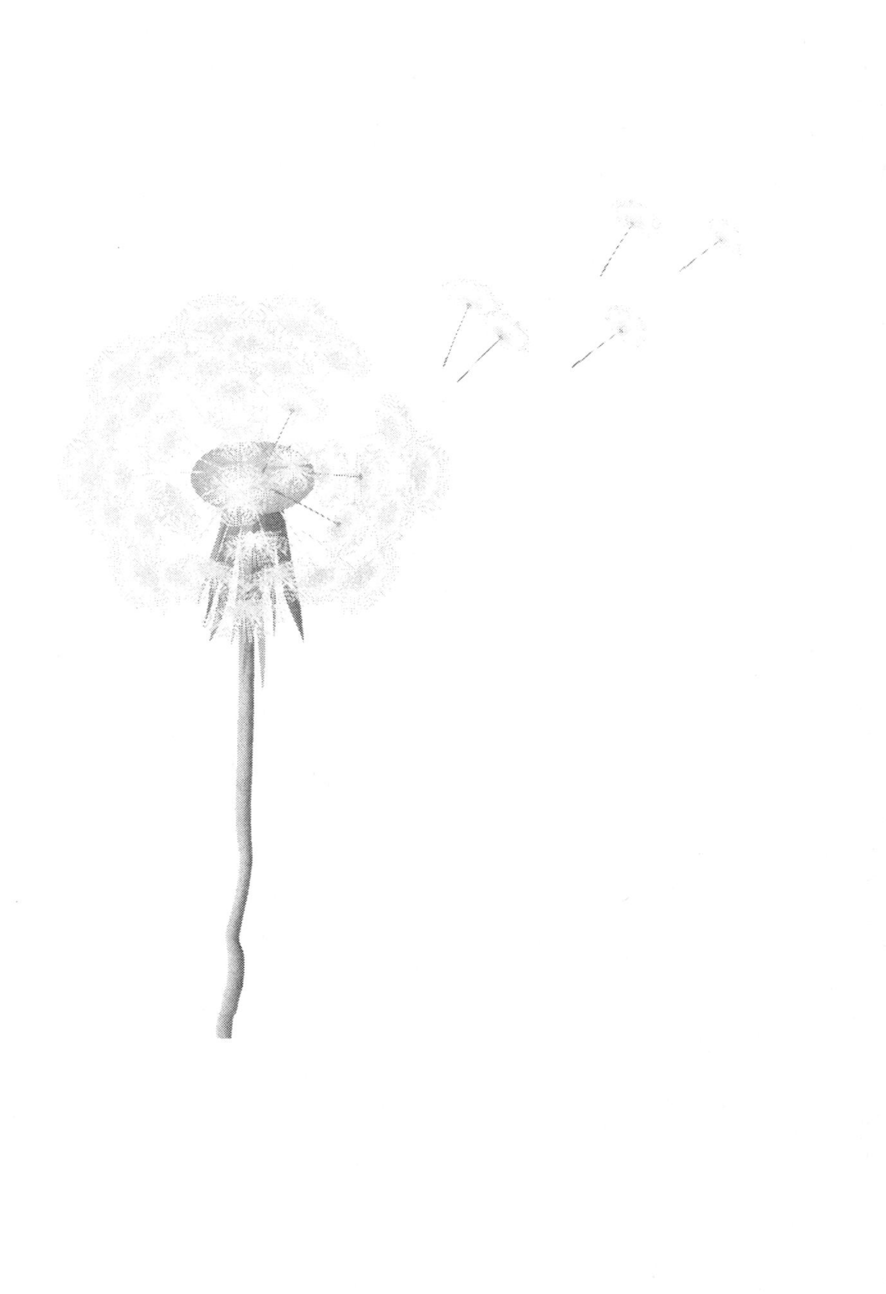

Faith

"You'll never believe what I did today. I got in the tub last night and I didn't trip!" This was her big news she wanted to share with me. And for this patient, it really *was* big news. Her cancer had spread to her brain, and the side effects of her chemotherapy had damaged some of her nerves and affected her balance. Little victories like successfully getting into a bathtub were great celebrations.

She bravely fought cancer for over 12 years. Whenever she faced a change in her disease, we had to clarify the findings with more tests, more scans. She was not anxious about needing additional tests. Instead, she would just nod calmly and say, "So, we just need more information that's all."

She reminded me so much of my mom. My mother and I escaped communism by immigrating to America from Yugoslavia. We arrived with a few suitcases of our belongings. We spoke only a few words of English—whatever we'd learned from watching *Bonanza* episodes on television, which we were surprised to learn were useless in New York City. We were poor and alone in our new country. But my mother had the uncanny ability to turn any situation around and look at it sharply from a positive perspective. My mother had been dead many years, but this patient reminded me of her. Neither one despaired or gave up hope when things turned bleak. They kept the faith. To someone like my mom, the blacker the night, the brighter the stars.

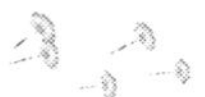

As the breast cancer spread to my patient's brain and liver and I felt she could not take one more setback, she developed tongue cancer. After surgery removed part of her tongue, one might think that would slow her down, but it never did. When I walked in her room, she smiled and burst into a beautifully garbled "alleluia" at the top of her weakened voice. She felt that having a part of her tongue remove was an effort to stop her from sharing her faith. It only made her try even harder to minister to others.

The nails on her fingers fell off, and the skin on her red, raw hands peeled severely as a side effect from treatment. She just covered the pain with cute flower-printed gardening gloves. She found great joy in the little things. I remember when she discovered that a frozen orange was just the right size and shape to soothe the burning sensation as she cupped her hands around it. I can still see the childlike grin on her face describing her discovery to me as if she had found treasure.

She made a lasting impression on everyone who knew her. (We still talk about her in my office today and even remember her birthday.) She talked to other patients receiving chemotherapy beside her, cultivating an unusual camaraderie in transient moments with people she might never see again. She was particularly attuned to others' needs and always looked for a "reason" behind everything that happened. One time when she was admitted to the hospital, she ministered to the woman who cleaned her room, once again gracefully bypassing the layers of superficiality that would normally keep two very different women apart. I'd seen my mother do the same thing many times with strangers, drawing out of them with ease what they'd never told another soul. Although my patient was released before she could complete her "mission," she happily picked up where she left off with the cleaning woman after being re-admitted a few months later!

No matter what came her way, she dealt with it in a spirit of graciousness. She could look at hopeless situations and envision some good in it somewhere. We, the medical community, saw it only one way: there was no cure for her. Even then, she found something that she could hang onto. She took time to write me encouraging little notes. She wrote that she was praying for me to get plenty of rest so I could make the best decision in each situation she faced. You'd think she'd spend all her time praying for herself and her own family. Not her—she intentionally prayed for others. Doctor and patient, we took care of each other.

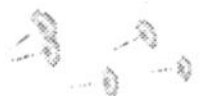

She progressively declined and moved to the Intensive Care Unit. She knew her days were numbered now, and she chose to live each one without being distracted by the fear of dying. One day, her son was playing his guitar and singing Christian praise songs for her in her room. She did not want any more treatment. This was how she wanted to go. My patient was happy going to another place—she was going home.

I've noticed that people of faith have less fear of dying. When death nears, there is some sense of relief to it. Patients associate cancer with loss. They lose their hair and parts of their body and often lose sight of who they are in the process. For some, death is a new beginning that will restore all that was taken from them.

I think faith is something that is shared between doctors and patients. As a doctor, I believe I can help anyone get to the other side of their journey. I don't promise a smooth ride to get there, and I let my patients lean on me when their hope fades. Patients need to decide what they're willing to live for—something in the future worth staying alive to see. For some, it's seeing a child grow up and graduate. For others, it's that moment when they walk their daughter down the aisle. I try to learn as much as I can about my patients so I can help them focus on what is important to them during the hard times. Sometimes a glimpse of better times in the future is all it takes to fight through difficulty now.

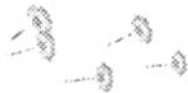

After my patient died, I was making my usual rounds in the hospital and saw a photograph in the hallway that reminded me of her. It was two rainbows—her favorite. I must have passed that photograph a thousand times before without noticing it, but since her death rainbows had more meaning for me. It was just like her—showing me one more time how to see what ordinarily could not be seen. She saw hope where some would say there was so little to hope for. And she had faith when it seemed so difficult to believe.

Faith is to believe what you do not see;
the reward of this faith is to see what you believe.
—Saint Augustine

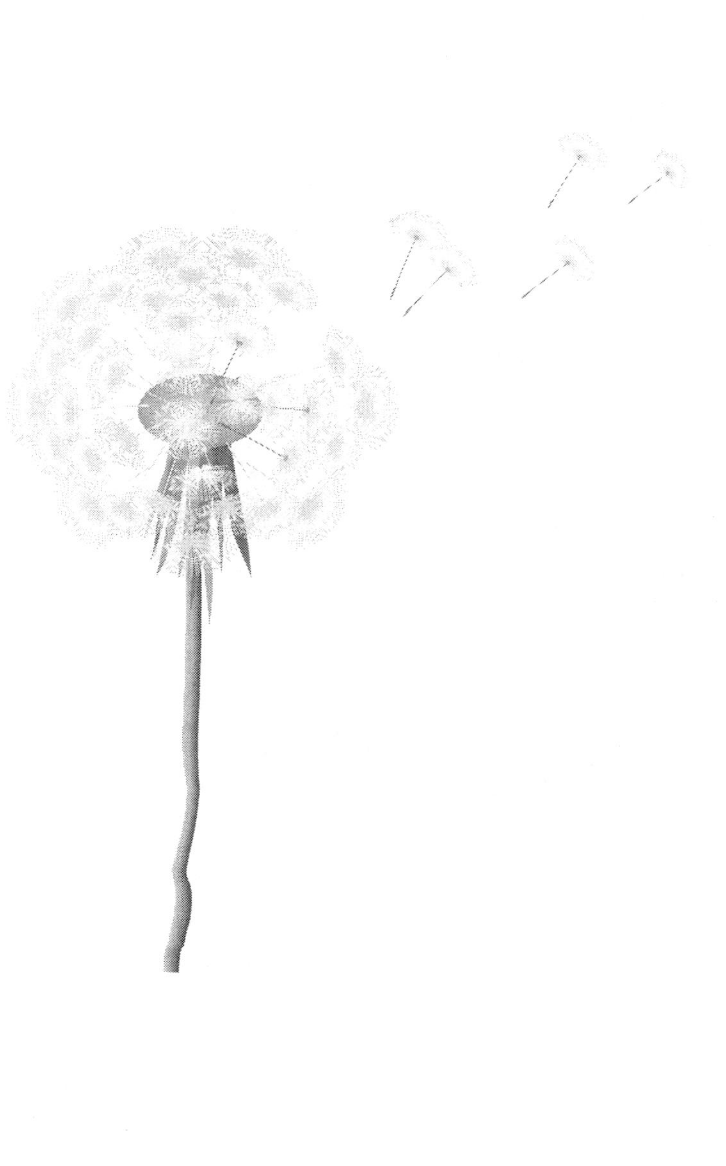

Kindness

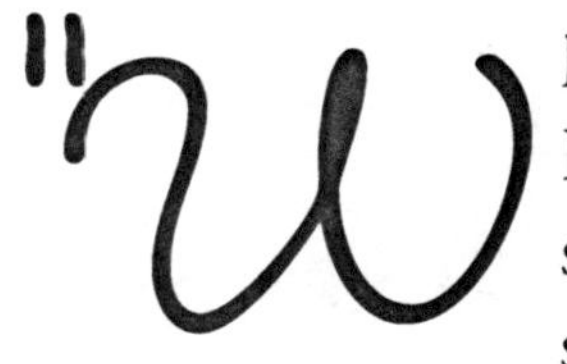

hat is that?" I said when I walked in her room and saw one wall covered with sticky-notes.

I was visiting a patient in the hospital whose chemotherapy treatment had lowered her white blood cell count. She needed to raise her blood count before she could be released home safely.

She needed 350 white blood cells to be specific.

She had asked me earlier to draw some white blood cells on a piece of paper. So, I sketched a few cells, not knowing what she would do with the drawing. Now there were 350 yellow sticky-note drawings of similar white blood cells on the wall of her hospital room. She was an artist and had drawn the young and mature white blood cells in detail.

As her white blood cell count increased, she removed that many sticky notes off the wall. Each note she peeled off meant she was one step closer to being discharged and sent home.

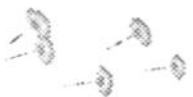

At first, I thought she was in shock—she was so calm about the whole process. Many patients are very stressed when they have to be hospitalized. Not this one. She just looked at the goal ahead and visualized getting better, removing the sticky notes one by one.

When you choose to live in the moment, as my artist patient did, you want to feel every bit of it. I think that's why she drew the white blood cells—she wanted to experience everything on the deepest, cellular level. You will rarely meet a more focused person than someone who is fighting against cancer. It's as if they shut down everything else in life that competes for their attention. They don't multi-task. The single priority is trying to stay alive. Every facet of life becomes intensely vivid, raw and real. They have only a finite amount of energy each day, and they don't want to waste it on trivial things.

When you choose to live like this—or even when you don't choose it and you're forced into it—your focus changes. Instead of denying the reality of cancer, you start incorporating that experience. Instead of life becoming much smaller, it suddenly becomes much bigger and greater than you ever imagined. I tell my patients, "Don't cheat yourself out of the journey that your life is taking you on."

But my life will never be the same! some will say.

"You're right. Your life will never be the same again," I tell them. "But it could be better." For many, cancer is forcing them to live...and not just exist.

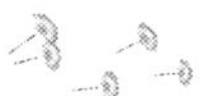

Everyone who is diagnosed with cancer is focused on recovery. *What will I need to do to recover from this?* That's understandable. But in being so focused on the end goal or destination, we can miss the journey along the way. When patients reach the end of treatment, some think, "Well, that's the end of that." I know people who recover and want to pretend the cancer never happened. But they cheat themselves out of discovering more of who they are *because* of cancer.

That is why it's more about discovery, not recovery, as this same patient showed me when she planned a weekend retreat for other cancer patients. She and I shared a belief in art as medicine, and we hoped painting, music and writing at a spa-like retreat would create an environment where patients could be pampered and process their emotions. Here, they discovered gifts they never knew they had.

There is so much more to us than even we know about ourselves. Cancer peels away the superficiality and brings people to the core of who they really are. Under certain circumstances in life, doors will open that were never opened before. We'll see what we've never seen and try what we've never tried. When we're scared of an unknown like cancer and chemotherapy, sometimes our imagination is much worse than the actual experience. Once patients push their initial fears to the edge, they are more open to exploring other unknown parts of themselves.

At the retreat, patients who were afraid to put anything on paper before began writing beautiful poetry about their experience. Patients who had never painted before began painting with their eyes closed, moved along by the music playing softly in the background. When they opened their eyes and saw their canvas, they were more amazed than we were. They discovered the artist within.

Because of what this patient has done for others, she represents the culmination of seeds patients have planted in my life: patience, hope, goodness, love, peace, faith—and especially kindness—all packaged together in grace. *What a kindness to help others discover who they are.* The seeds she continues to plant in others' lives today have made their lives better tomorrow.

Everybody can be great because everybody can serve.
You only need a heart full of grace...you can be that servant.
—Martin Luther King, Jr.

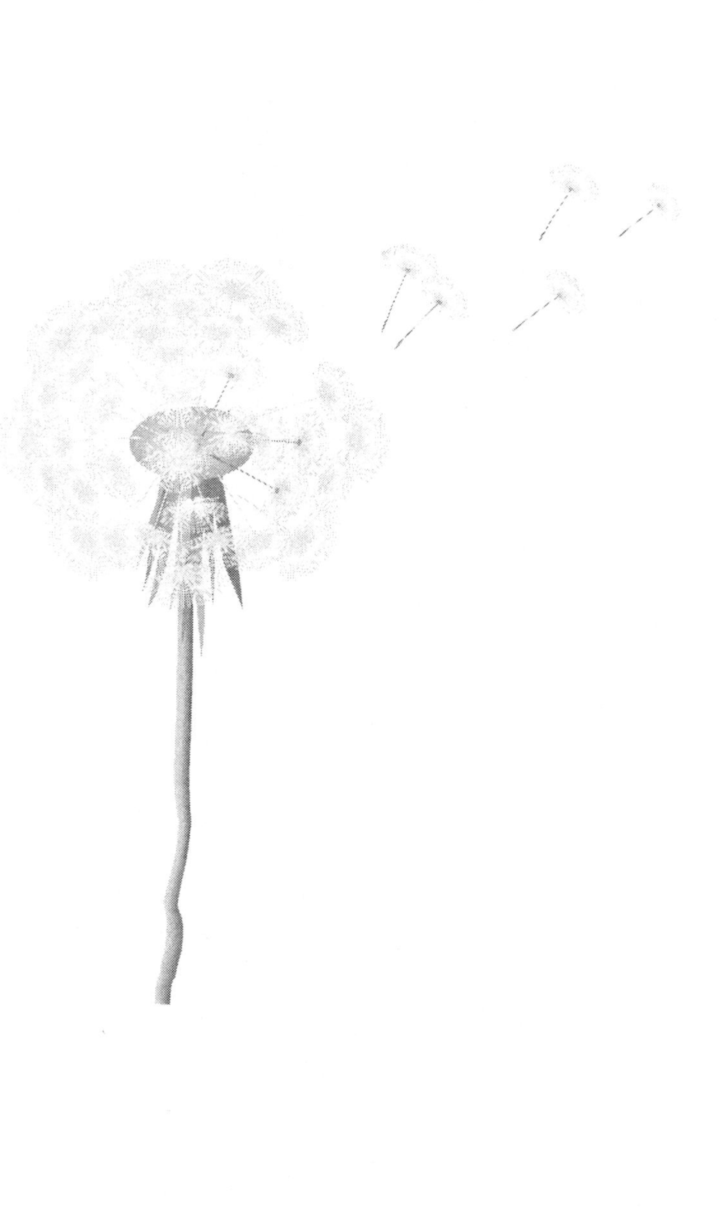

Prayer

"Why are you crying?"

The computer tech who was working on my office computer had tears in his eyes. It was the end of the day and he still hadn't fixed it. "It's okay, alright?" I told him. "You can just come back tomorrow to finish—don't get so upset!"

"That's just it...I can't finish tomorrow," he said, wiping his eyes. "My mother-in-law is sick, and we're renting out a movie theater tomorrow so she can watch *Toy Story 3* without disturbing anyone because she coughs."

This piqued my interest. "She's that sick? What does she have?" He told me she'd had an uncontrollable cough and pain in her shoulder for years. "I think she has breast cancer, but we don't know," he said.

"You *think* she has breast cancer?" I said. "Either she does or she doesn't...has she ever been diagnosed?"

No. She had not.

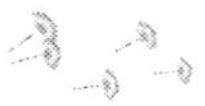

The reason she had not been diagnosed is because she and her pastor husband were praying that God would heal her apart from traditional medicine. They had never seen a doctor. No X-rays. And certainly no biopsies. She was not afraid of dying—she was just patiently waiting for God to determine when her time was up. When I learned that she had lived with this "condition" for years, I knew we could probably do something to help her. But how, if she would not let us?

I told the son-in-law to ask if she would let me come see her in her home. This was the first of all the miracles that happened in her story because he asked her—and she agreed. So, my husband and I traveled to another town to visit her at home three days later. Suspecting the diagnosis would most certainly be breast cancer, I brought some things along with me, including some sample medicines for nausea and breast cancer hormone therapies that I thought might help. *If she will not come to the doctor, let the doctor go to her* I thought.

Her husband met us at the door, and I could tell he was skeptical. But, he let us in. His wife was sitting in a recliner in her housecoat, coughing and holding her right shoulder in considerable pain. She was pale, very weak and her eyes were dull. We talked for a while about her history, but I was still unsure if she would let me examine her. I discovered she was an artist and art teacher. Her husband showed us her small art studio next to the living room. She thought she had broken something in her arm or shoulder and could no longer teach or paint because of the pain. She had sold her car, told her relatives goodbye and now she was waiting to die. She felt the end that she had been praying for was finally near.

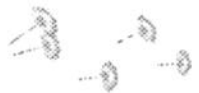

I had been praying on the way to her home that it would be obvious that her complaints were tied to her breast. I was hoping for a visible skin lesion or something that would make a strong case for treating her for breast cancer without having a biopsy. I assumed that was out of the question. Meanwhile, her husband was a devout man of God who had also been praying. He wanted God to perform a miracle—and that's exactly what his wife needed. She needed a miracle. Knowing he was a faithful and godly man, I wanted to honor his prayers and not insult him. So, I asked him: "What if your prayers have been answered? You've been wanting a miracle. Not only did you not have to take her to the doctor; the doctor came to you! If that's not a miracle, I don't know what is."

After we talked a while longer, he finally allowed me to examine her. When I removed the dressing covering an open wound near her collarbone and breast, it was immediately clear she had breast cancer. Untreated, it had spread toward her shoulder. Thankfully, she was willing to take the hormone medicine I had brought. When I examined her again weeks later, her response was dramatic. After years of pain, the ulceration near her shoulder had healed, and she was gaining strength every day. She proudly told me she had painted her kitchen ceiling using her right hand, not minding that it took her three days to finish. And she even bought a new car!

Now, she could dress without pain, paint and teach her art classes again. Her first painting after her recovery was for me. She named it *Serenity Lane* because of the new path she now traveled—a peaceful, tree-lined path leading to future possibilities. What happened to her did not negate their faith—it reinforced it. And now they are able to share their story with others in their circles of influence with similar reservations about doctors and medicine. (She even jokes with her husband that if he misbehaves she will cremate him and put his urn in a doctor's office!)

She thanks God for the scar on her collarbone because it is in an area she doesn't mind showing to others as evidence of her healing. She is spreading her own seeds through her powerful story of how God worked to heal her through prayer and traditional medicine. It could not be a coincidence because I did not even know she existed three days prior. And, I later learned, her husband would never have let me examine her if I were a male doctor. I was a woman, a person of faith and an artist myself. Only God could line up all these factors to save her life. Her healing was a gift from God and a strong message for other patients who are reluctant to consider traditional medical treatment.

Prayer and conventional medicine can go hand in hand. When you pray for help and God sends it, you should take it. Prayer is the only treatment that does not have any potential negative side effects—no nausea, no hair loss. There is no insurance coding for prayer, and there is no need for any special equipment or place to do it—it is free and accessible to everyone. Prayer treats the entire person (body, soul, mind and spirit).

Best of all, it works.

When you pray for help and God sends it,
you should take it.

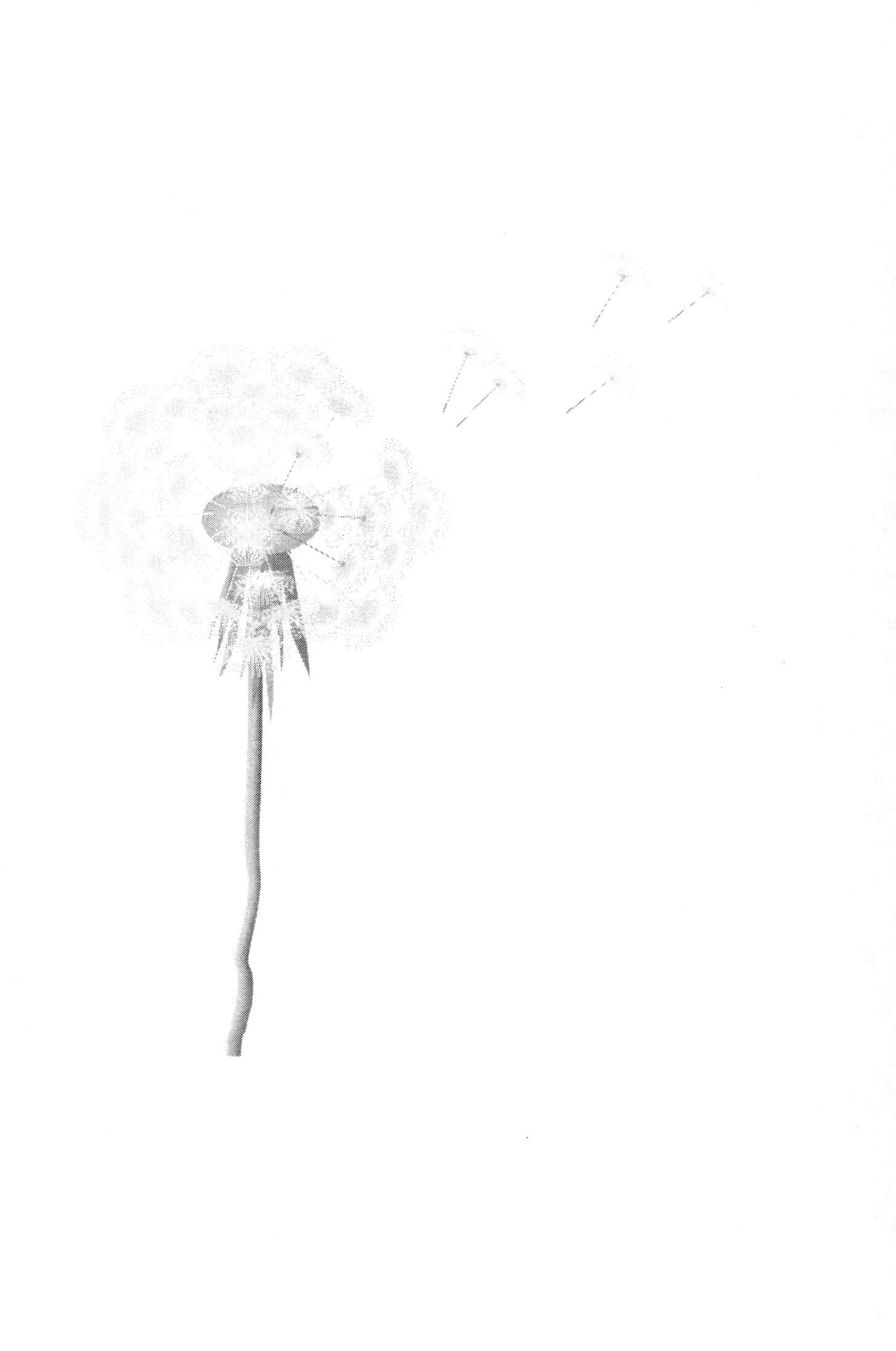

Giving

Her bucket list was very short. She knew her remaining time on earth was limited. She just wanted to help one other woman. And continue to paint.

When I first met her, she lived alone in a very humble home, enjoyed a simple lifestyle and mowed her own grass. She surrounded herself with the things she loved: family photos, her cat, lots of knickknacks and her brushes, paints and her easel. Her paintings covered nearly every wall surface. Some pieces were framed and many were not, much like my mother who painted on anything that was not nailed down. "Nothing is sacred and everything is a potential canvas," as my mother had often said.

But she spent hours each afternoon using a sleeve compression machine to help relieve some of the pressure in her swollen, achy arm. Her cancer was gone, but prior surgery and radiation had left one arm permanently swollen.

This was the arm that would change lives, starting with her own.

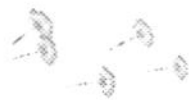

I visited her on Sundays when she finally moved to assisted living. My daughter was a child then, and we often laughed at her skipping down the hall to the cafeteria in a lunchtime "race" against other residents slowly hobbling along the wall. She and her friend were always ready to put on an impromptu show of singing and dancing, too.

Back in her room after sharing a meal, the compression routine began as she settled into her blue recliner. While my daughter played with her cat, I listened to her stories over the constant humming from the compressor, a time machine transporting us to another time and place where she was a young girl again with her sister and mother.

She taught me that you don't have to have a lot in order to give to someone else. No one could have guessed that she had a longstanding dream to build a state-of-the-art breast care center. Years ago, she had discovered a mass in her breast, but she waited several months before seeing a doctor. Where should she go? She was lost and alone. After her treatment and recovery, she promised herself that no other woman would feel the way she had felt.

Today, the breast cancer center that she envisioned is named after her and is a leading facility for breast cancer screening and intervention. It is located in the building where I work, but it feels much more like walking into her living room. (Only now the paintings are all framed, and a few of her favorite knickknacks that used to be scattered around her home are neatly arranged in a glass cabinet.)

Sometimes I think she might walk in at any moment, her hands covered with dried paint from painting at her easel, and welcome everyone waiting for a mammogram. Thankfully, she was able to attend the facility's grand opening and see it while she was alive. I also have a photo of her wearing a pink Race for the Cure t-shirt from one of those early breast cancer awareness events she helped us host.

My friend's bad arm changed her life as an artist because it interfered with her work. She even told me once that she chose her clothes based on what best fit around her arm. But that same arm also changed lives for the better. The constant reminder made her realize how many others were affected daily by the same disease, and it motivated her to do something about it.

She didn't want to change the world. She often told me, "If I can only help one person, it will be worth it." Mother Teresa once said of her own work among the poor in India, "We ourselves feel that what we are doing is just a drop in the ocean. But the ocean would be less because of that missing drop."

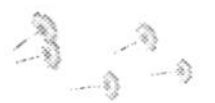

Every time a patient chooses to use their own demise for the good of others it reminds me of a seed. It doesn't seem like much at first. You *don't* have to have much in order to give. It may be a small sacrifice or a tiny kindness. One seed doesn't require a lot either. You water it and wait (sometimes a long time) for it to grow. However, when it grows, the results are exponential. Not knowing that she would eventually help thousands, it was the attempt to help just one that made all the difference. It mattered to that one.

Anyone can count the seeds in an apple,
but only God can count the number of apples in a seed.
—Robert H. Schuller

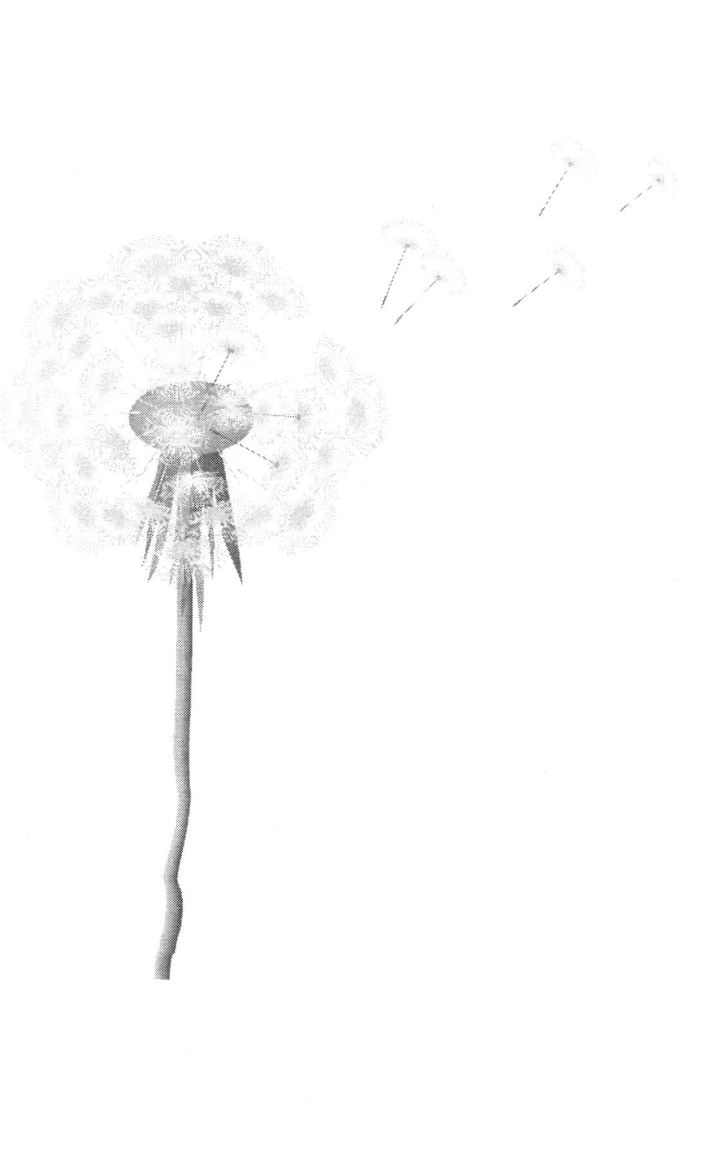

Patience

It was a busy day, busier than usual with several emergencies.

My nurse told me my new patient had been waiting in the exam room for a long while. I was on my way to see him when someone burst out of the door and started briskly walking down the hall toward the exit.

Is this my patient? I wondered as I followed him out into the hall, the clickety-clack sound of his cowboy boots slapping the tile. He was walking so quickly that I didn't catch up with him until he was nearly in the parking lot. "Sir, are you my new patient?" I asked.

"Not anymore," he said tight-lipped. "I have better things to do than wait..."

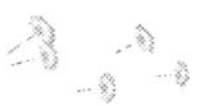

I could tell he was tense and angry. I told him, "I am very sorry for keeping you waiting. I would like for you to meet me first and then you can decide if you want to be my patient or not."

After a moment, he agreed to come back inside. When we reached the exam room, I started asking him my typical questions about family history. I learned he had a strong family history of heart disease and high blood pressure. His blood pressure was high that day. I mentioned that people sometimes die sooner from these medical conditions than from cancer! We connected that day, and I've enjoyed taking care of him as a patient since then. I even joked with him that waiting for his appointments would be part of his therapy so he could relax and learn to be patient. And he did. Later, he told me that chasing him down in the parking lot was not "crazy"! It showed him how much I cared.

He reminded me of Kenny Rogers with his white hair and trimmed beard. He had been diagnosed with breast cancer, which is much less common in men. It all started when he was getting out of the shower one day and his wife (who is a nurse) noticed one of his nipples was inverted, which can be an indication of breast cancer. And it was. He completed his treatment and is still cancer-free.

In fact, after he shared his story with some local publications, several men contacted him about their own experience with breast cancer. By talking about the risk of breast cancer in males, he may have even saved their lives. When his mother later received her own cancer diagnosis, he helped guide her through it.

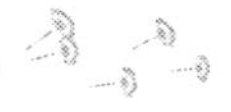

Cancer does not fit into a busy life. It is inconvenient, expensive, and it creates more work for everyone involved. Going to the doctor is often the last item on everyone's list, especially men. As my patient discovered, cancer moves your health to the top of the list and rearranges your priorities.

Cancer has the potential to teach us more about patience and living moment to moment than perhaps any other life experience. You cannot make plans when you are undergoing treatment. For example, my patients receive a schedule when they begin treatment, but it is tentative. After their first cycle, patients often ask me if the next one will be the same. Perhaps. Perhaps not. We may have to alter it to get the results we want. Just when we get used to something in life, we often find ourselves back in uncertainty again.

Cancer forces you to slow down, but it also creates its own kind of busyness and preoccupation with side effects and appointments. I see patients who recover and actually experience separation anxiety from the clinic. They became so busy trying not to die that they forgot how to live when it's over. A lot of literature is devoted to helping patients come to grips with this new reality when their last treatment ends. They don't know whether to laugh or cry because they're just now processing what happened to them. My job is to help them never lose their identity in the first place and help them process the new realization that they are going to be okay.

People don't like to deal with uncertainty. I know I don't like it. I would like to get rid of cancer today or at least in my lifetime. However, waiting is inherent to the experience of cancer. And not just for the patients, for the doctors too. When I introduce a new treatment to a patient, we must wait to see what side effects they will experience and what benefit they will obtain. When I order follow up scans, we're waiting on the images to show a change. Everyone is different, and every cycle of treatment is different. Lots of uncertainty. Cancer treatment demands a steady pace from everyone involved.

Life is uncertain. We pretend that life happens on schedule, but our existence on earth is actually very transient. I encourage patients to take it one day at a time. Once patients learn to take shorter steps, their vision becomes extraordinarily crisp and defined "in the moment." That's why most patients can remember the exact time and date when they were diagnosed because the details are imprinted in their memories.

Others are so far out from their diagnosis that they barely remember it.

As time goes on, that defining moment settles into their lives and blends with the rest of who they are. Cancer becomes a part of their life, just another experience. There are no good or bad experiences, just experiences. The summation of all those makes us who we are.

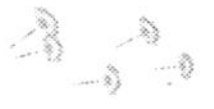

I think of battling cancer like driving in dense fog. We don't see the entire path but only what's directly ahead of us. If we successfully navigate what is in front of us, then the next part comes into view. And the next part after that. It's the "what ifs" about what we can't see that distract us from really *feeling* and paying attention to each step right now. Today's certainty gives us strength to face tomorrow's unknown.

This patient's story reminds me that we can all learn to wait and still get to where we ultimately want to be. While we are in a holding pattern, we must continue to live. Some of my patients just exist from one doctor visit to the next, instead of living between them. They hold their breath between check-ups, hoping for one more good report.

Contrast that with another patient I knew whose cancer gave her limited time. We customized her chemotherapy treatment when she asked to have three weeks off between treatments instead of two. "I have to have time to live. I need travel time. And time with the people I love," she informed us. She was in charge of her life, and her treatment would have to accommodate. A sharply dressed woman, she was always color-coordinated with the seasons. She was once late to an appointment with me because she lost an earring and stopped to buy new ones so would still look her best. Christmas was her favorite time of the year, and she took herself off her treatment to enjoy it. That Christmas was her last and her best.

*"If you worry today about tomorrow,
you will spoil both of them."*

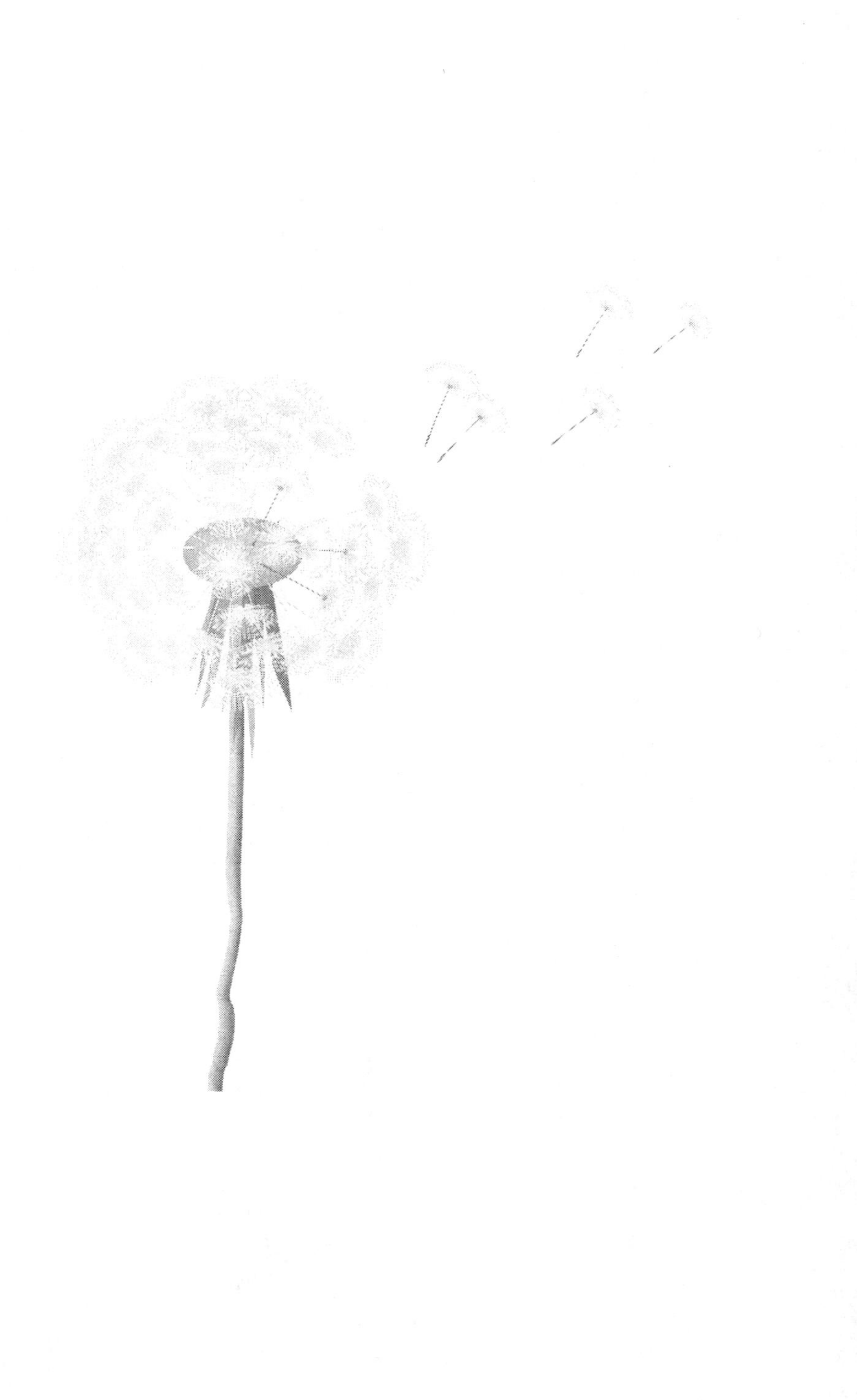

Hope

She was dying.

That's when she asked me if I was better off knowing her as a friend than not knowing her at all. At that moment, I was hurting so much because I was in the process of losing her: my patient and my friend. But she had this persistently hopeful smile on her face—so girlish as always. Her eyes twinkled as she laid her bald head against the pillow of her hospital bed and waited for my answer.

Yes, I decided. I was better off knowing her even for a short while.

I'd always felt a connection to my patients. However, after this particular patient died, I made a conscious decision to let down my barriers between my patients and me. I did not want it to be *Us—the physicians,* versus *Them—the patients*. We are all potential patients; some of us just haven't been diagnosed yet. If we work together as a team in the fight against cancer, everyone will be better off. I've always believed it was possible to become a better person inside even when your physical body is outwardly deteriorating. That was this patient's story. And I'll never forget her.

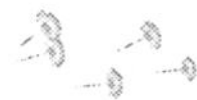

They were all sucking on bright orange popsicles when I walked into the hospital room that day. *"Oh, I have to get a picture of this,"* I said to myself. Her young son and daughter were snuggled up beside their mother in the bed, sharing the orange paisley pillowcase she'd brought from home. It was the perfect picture of contentment. She was happy and feeling good, fighting so hard to protect her children from what was happening.

Their fresh orange lips curled into smiles when I snapped the photo—how we all wished we could freeze life right then and enjoy it forever. She raised her hand weakly and welcomed me into the moment they were sharing. I slowed down enough to mentally erase whatever stress I'd carried into the room from my visits with other patients, and I realized something. I realized that the saying on the front of a t-shirt she often wore was true: life *is* good. It really is.

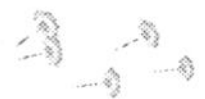

She was a person of "unmatched goodness," as one of her friends described her. She was the best mom. I remember going to a birthday party she had hosted for her son when she was feeling better. I took my daughter since they went to school together. She had hidden little objects throughout the house and also buried some in the sandbox outside in the yard for the children to find in a mini-scavenger hunt. They "panned" for gold, sifting through sand to find tiny gold specks. She even made a volcano cake that spewed red lava down the sides. (I still don't know how she did that!). I felt so sad to lose a friend—and even more sad that her children would not know a great mom like her for a longer period of time. But she was trying to build memories to last them a lifetime.

She wanted her children to know what was happening to Mommy so they would not be afraid. I remember her son came with her to an appointment one day, and she told me he had a question for me. "Sure," I said. "What do you want to know?" He shoved his little hand into the front pocket of his khaki school uniform pants and pulled out a wadded up piece of paper. "Where does the cancer come from?" he read aloud. I thought, "What a good question."

I began talking with him and even took him to the lab with me so we could look at some slides of blood cells. On his next visit with his mom, I called him over to me before she went in for her chemo treatment and put a sticky toy eyeball in his palm that I'd bought at a costume shop. "I'll keep an eye on your mom," I said as I pointed to the eyeball. It was a fun way to assure kids that when their mom came for her chemotherapy appointments she would be safe in my care. That always made them smile.

She was frustrated by the lack of information about cancer told from a child's viewpoint to help her own kids and other families. One day she told me she decided to create a book. I introduced her to another patient, an artist, who happened to be there that morning. They made a rough draft of the book within two weeks: *Mom Has Cancer: What do I do?* The book would help other children understand cancer in a non-frightening way through games and activities. It had a fun maze that "connected" Mommy to her chemotherapy, and children could also color different wigs and hats on a drawing of a Mommy without any hair. They even included tips about how to help Mommy around the house, letting her nap more and being sure to wash their hands frequently.

It was a book for kids, by kids because we let our own young children illustrate it. A pharmaceutical company printed the book for us and distributed it for free around the country, packaged with a box of 12 crayons. It was a great book for children who needed help understanding what was happening to their mom.

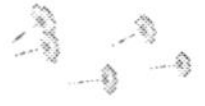

My patient had been looking forward to taking her daughter to her first day of school all summer. It was fall now. The leaves were starting to change and so was her prognosis. We both knew her last wish might not come true—she might be too ill to leave her bed even for a short while. With some help from others, we wheeled her down the corridor, out the back door and into my waiting car. All the while, I worried that she might collapse or have a seizure because she was on such a high dose of morphine for pain. But we made it to the first day of school.

She never stopped smiling, her eyes sparkling beneath the brim of a tan hat covering her bald head.

Her daughter seemed innocently unaware of the sacrifice her mom had made. To her, Mom would always be there beside her on her first day of school. *Where else would she be if she could possibly help it?* Her mom touched the chair she would sit in that year and tucked her new backpack into the cubby that had her name on it. Then she grazed her thin, pale hand across the top of her desk as if trying to feel every part of where her daughter would be that year and somehow mark it with her touch.

As the other families milled around, she asked her daughter to sit behind her desk so she could take a mental snapshot of her little girl sitting there and store it in her memory. I imagined she would go to that simple schoolroom scene a dozen times in her mind later that afternoon, trying with great difficulty to remember every detail despite the "morphine fog" wiping them away one by one. When we returned to the hospital and I asked her if she'd had a good day, she simply said, "It was awesome."

So, whenever I think of her I often picture the orange popsicle day. I remember a cleaning man was nearby playing a mandolin in the break room. I asked him if he would please play for them. It was surreal. But at the same time, seeing this stranger playing softly in the background as her kids enjoyed what would be one of their last moments with their mom reminded me that this was worth it. It was worth it to let my guard down and let them inside my heart. It was worth it to hold onto hope—and the beautiful gift of friendship—when everything else loses meaning. When we put a "cancer bell" in a park gazebo for survivors to ring, she had said it was "perfect." I asked her why she thought so. She said, "Because *hope rings eternal.*" And so it does.

Love recognizes no barriers. It jumps hurdles, leaps fences, penetrates walls to arrive at it destination full of hope.

—Maya Angelou

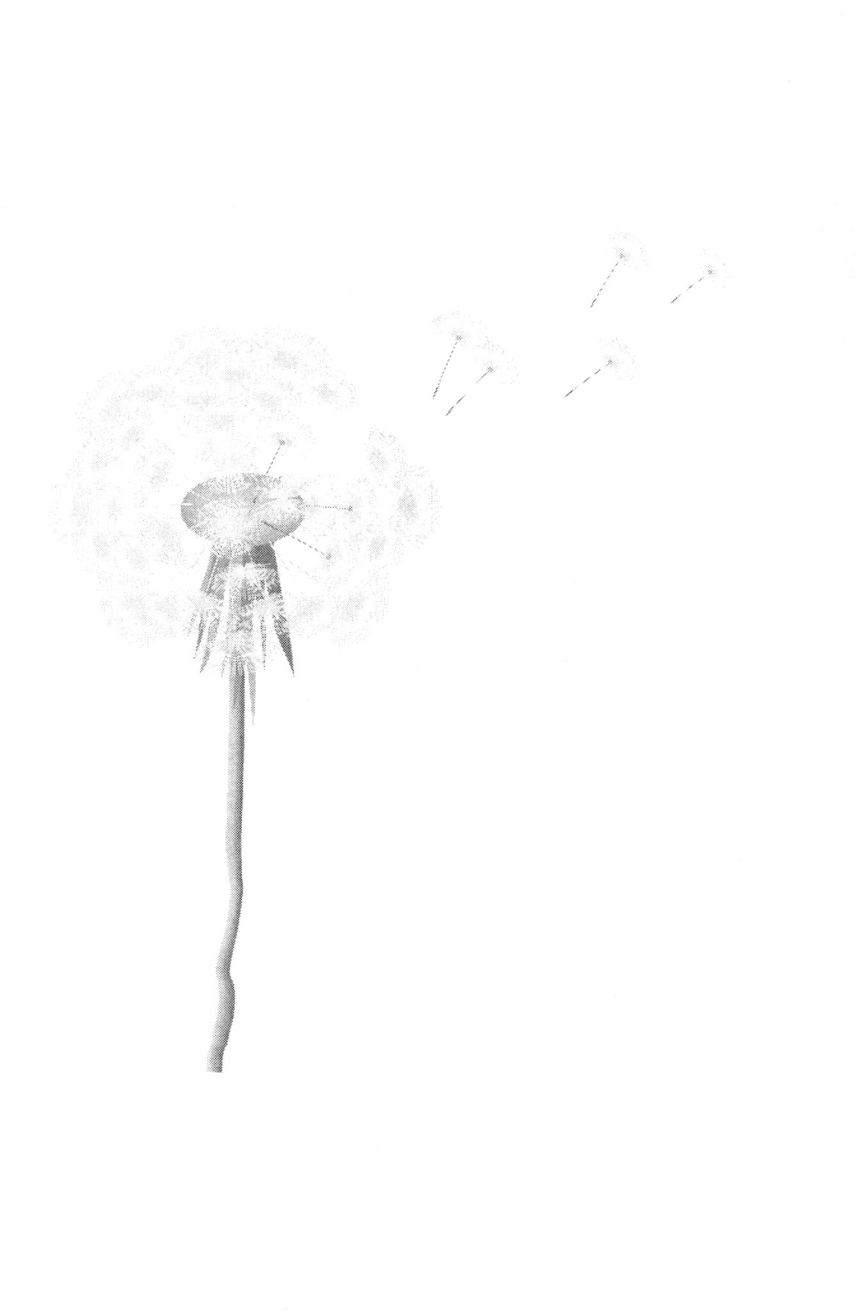

Joy

It was Tuesday.

Another Field Trip Day. That's what we called them. On my day off, we would have adventures together. I remember we would pack a lunch and just go somewhere—anywhere.

She introduced me to cucumber sandwiches. Never heard of them. The crispy cucumbers and cream cheese on grain bread was so good that I can almost taste it right now. She loved it when she could teach me something new, something American.

Sometimes we would just frame paintings that we had painted. We read jokes, although she found it much more amusing than the jokes themselves whenever I didn't get the punch lines. (Humor doesn't always translate across cultures. Ask me to tell you a Yugoslavian joke sometime.)

Her friendship was so dear to me. Although she was my patient, we hardly ever talked about her cancer outside of the clinic. Time was short. Instead of helping her, her treatments were giving her more side effects. We knew the cancer was there, growing inside of her. Yet there were so many other beautiful distractions around us to talk about instead.

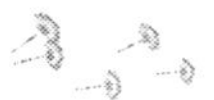

Even when she wanted to talk about it, she would stop herself, and we would turn our attention to the bright colors of her newest painting. When she got a new roof on her house, she saved the old slate tiles. "What are you going to do with all these?" I asked her one day, pointing to the boxes of tiles. With a sparkle in her eye, she answered, "We're going to *paint* them!"

We loaded up the boxes and took them to a local art place for children so they could paint on them. They painted all kinds of things on them—splashing color onto the lifeless grey slate. Then they took her tiles home with them, spreading seeds of her love for art all over town.

She wrote little stories about her paintings to document what inspired a particular work. One time she was waiting on a giftwrapped purchase at a department store and saw a painting on the wall behind her that prompted her to do a whole series of paintings. We hung many of her pieces in the Chemo Gallery where patients receive treatment. Her journey through life was colorful, and the hues and combinations of textures she used for her art brightened the atmosphere for patients who were in an otherwise dark place physically and emotionally.

Knowing there was only so much life left made her live to the fullest every day. The dark thunderclouds were on their way. In the meantime, she would add extra colors to life's everyday colors in everything from her paintings to her wardrobe. When she painted, she made the blue sky bluer and the sunshine brighter than I've ever seen.

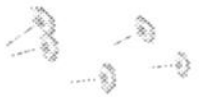

One of her favorite things to do was to show up for her appointments dressed in costume. In football season, she wore a Cheese Head (a yellow rubber triangle hat that Green Bay Packer fans wear). Another time, I opened the door to the exam room to see a three-foot tall pink bouffant wig piled on her head. "You did not tell me about all the side-effects," she said, trying not to smile. I ran and got my camera. Another time, she came as a Geisha girl because she knew we were hosting Chinese missionary doctors in our home that week. She'd painted her face white, and she bowed and shuffled her way to the exam room. My staff just laughed! They looked forward to her visits to see what she would do next. She loved life and embraced all of it.

My patient was the queen of the unexpected, and her spontaneity often showed up in her artwork. She painted every imaginable kind of frog, a reminder of her favorite acronym: F.R.O.G. (Fully Rely On God). She painted a butterfly one time, its colorful wings spilling over from the edge of the canvas to the matte and even the frame. Life was too small a stage to contain someone like her. She spread her wings just like that butterfly and graced all those around her with amazing beauty.

Closer to my mother's age, she considered age just a number because she was so youthful and playful at heart. She put an exclamation point on every experience and raised it to the next notch. At her home, she put a whimsical sculpture of giant yellow daffodils in the front yard that bloom year around. I was driving around her neighborhood before we'd even met and noticed them one day. I drove up in their circle driveway to get a closer look and saw her husband standing outside. I introduced myself as a new cancer doctor in town (hoping he didn't mind that I was in his driveway!). "My wife has breast cancer," he told me, and that was the start of our friendship. After she died, he was also diagnosed with cancer. Now it was *his* turn to fight; and he did. Their grandson continued the fight for others by entering medical school.

"I want to do something for you," his wife said one day, wanting to thank me somehow for taking care of her. "Just be my friend," I told her. "The only gift I want is your friendship...and for you to paint your journey for me." One time, she painted the initial "V" out of a line of green apples on a black and white checkerboard background, a key lime forming the period. I still treasure it.

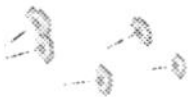

When the rain clouds finally came, she went home. I know heaven is a brighter place today because of her.

Life is not about waiting for the storm to pass.
It's about dancing in the rain.

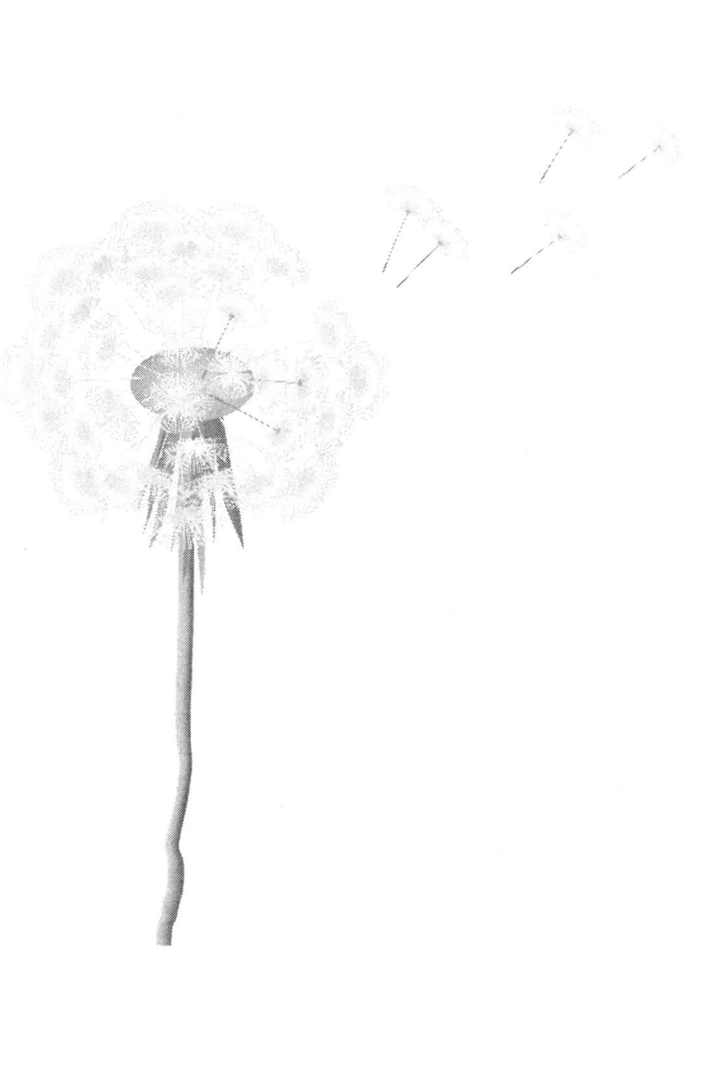

Endurance

No one had ever seen her with her clothes off.

No one.

She wouldn't even let me examine her with the lights on. For her first few appointments, I turned off the overhead lights and tried using only the dim under-cabinet lighting to examine her.

At the end of several months of treatment, I walked in the exam room one day to find her sitting there uncovered with the bright ceiling lights on. What a change! "Are you cold?" I asked her, trying not to seem overly surprised as I helped her into an examining gown. She just shrugged. "No, why do you ask?"

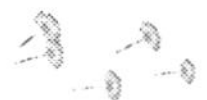

Her story reminds me that we all have something we have to get past or get over in order to make it. I could tell hundreds of stories about what I've learned from my patients about surviving. (My mom was an excellent storyteller who could entertain people with her broken English for hours. She made up for the words she didn't know by talking with her hands.) No two patient stories are alike because no one experiences cancer exactly the same way. Cancers are different. Treatments are different. Nevertheless, everyone makes the same discovery: they can handle far more than they ever thought they could.

Cancer changes everything. It changes your body, your appearance and most of your relationships. It lowers your defenses and breaks down your walls. It makes you fight. There are two responses to difficulty: give up or learn to fight. My mom taught me to fight (although she was so optimistic that I never realized that's what we were doing). At times in my childhood, we were often homeless, poor and even imprisoned—but we endured.

"Sasha, we have to do what we have to do now, so one day we can do what we want to do," she always told me. Some who know my personal story tell me I "inspire" them. It's the patient who continues to work and sing praises to the Lord, all the while battling cancer, who inspires me. It's the ones who tell me, "Cancer is a blessing in my life." The ones who say, "I have to stay alive for my kids." Those are the ones who inspire me.

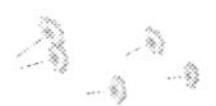

Patients use different techniques to help them endure difficulty. Visualization, for example, can be a very powerful tool. One patient told me he envisioned his tumor as a sand castle being washed away with each wave of chemotherapy. When he received his last treatment, he smiled and said confidently, "The sand castle is gone." Another patient pictured Pac-Man eating all the cancer in her body like the video game, clearing it away piece by piece.

Many of my patients consider laughter the best medicine. "Laughter is my kind of exercise," one of my patients told me. Laughing is like inner jogging; it keeps our souls in shape. Studies have shown that laughing actually releases endorphins that make you feel better. Wherever some of my patients see humor, I welcome it. One patient let her grandkids shave her thinning hair into a mohawk. When her hair fell out completely, they turned to sticking temporary-tattoos of Winnie the Pooh's Tigger on her bald head. Seeing an orange tattoo tiger playing tennis across her pink scalp and doing his best to cover the surgical scars from her double mastectomy, you could not help but laugh.

Another patient drew a big yellow smiley face on the back of her head. "Don't Worry. Be Happy," she added in big letters. A mother and daughter used to dress alike in funny costumes for the mom's weekly chemotherapy treatments. A little humor goes a long way when you see two grown women dressed as chickens in the treatment room!

One patient decided to get different wigs after her hair fell out. She bought a sassy red one, a long brown one, a short black one—all reflecting different personalities. She said that her husband never knew who he was going to bed with each night! Other patients try to outdo each other by wearing all pink, mismatched socks or carrying funky purses to their treatments. One of my patients wore a clever t-shirt after her surgery and reconstruction. The bold letters across her chest read, "Yes, they are fake. My real ones almost killed me."

Not everyone deals with difficulty the same way. I've seen a spectrum of reactions from patients over the years. When I served as a public health officer in New York City as part of medical school summer training, a hysterical woman called 911 to report that she had "cut off" her finger. The EMS personnel and I climbed seven stories to her apartment to discover that only the tiniest tip of her finger was actually missing. That same night, we responded to a call where a robber had shoved a woman through a store window and stolen her purse. When we arrived, the victim was running down the street after the guy with bloody shards of glass still sticking out of her back!

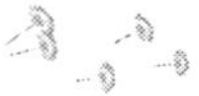

Sometimes my patients have already been through so much in life when they visit me for the first time. One patient with early breast cancer refused to take curative chemotherapy. She was deathly afraid of vomiting. She seemed completely paralyzed by fear at the thought of it. No one likes to experience nausea and vomiting, but her reaction was sheer terror.

I could not understand why she would refuse this treatment with two young kids who needed their mother to stay alive. She would live if she took the treatment, but she would most certainly die without it. I called her every day. I reassured her I could manage her nausea. I was even willing to put her in the hospital under heavy sedation to minimize the side effects. She did not want any part of it.

I talked to the psychiatrist on our oncology team about this patient because it was such an unusual case. I felt there was something we weren't seeing or understanding. He explained that traumatic experiences early in life can sometimes affect our decisions later on, without our being aware of it. In order to dig deeper in her subconscious and find out why she had such strong feelings about vomiting, he suggested hypnosis. When she agreed to be hypnotized, I was amazed. Even *she* knew that her response was inappropriate, and she wanted to know why. Afterwards, we talked about her session.

Under hypnosis, she had kneeled on the floor in the psychiatrist's office like a child. Shaking uncontrollably, she started scooping up imaginary material and rapidly shoving it in her mouth. She was screaming and saying, "I'm so sorry, Daddy. I'm so sorry." She had reverted to a childhood memory where her father had made her eat her own vomit when she accidentally threw up in his new car. She vowed that she would never vomit again. After recognizing the source of her fear, she agreed to go forward with standard treatment. I hospitalized her, and she successfully completed her treatment without vomiting.

I learned from this patient that our past experiences shape and direct our daily decisions. Although hypnosis is an extreme example, we need to dig deep inside to find out why we think the way we think. Some patients make decisions based on the experience of others. They will not want to undergo treatment because someone they knew had chemotherapy "and they died anyway." It's my job to sort that out so that when patients refuse treatment, we all need to understand why. It is a patient's right to decline treatment, but I hope the decision is not based on misinformation or the wrong reasons.

One of the strongest patients I'll never forget was ill for 10 years. She was so determined that she worked throughout her illness, even two days before she died. She told me early on that she desperately wanted to have a second child. We worked to help her stay healthy enough to finally get pregnant and carry a beautiful baby boy to term. When she died years later, this young man came to my office with his dad and thanked me for "having my mom as long as I did."

One day I was opening the mail at home when I saw a graduation announcement from the daughter of one of my patients. My husband looked over my shoulder and said the daughter was his patient at his dermatology practice. "Her mom was *my* patient," I said, thinking back to a conversation many years ago when a young mom with a young child wanted to live long enough to see her daughter graduate. That day was finally here. Later, I learned that unbeknownst to us her daughter was also the recipient of a scholarship that my husband and I had established. It was proof to me that endurance has its own reward. Don't give up too soon. There are many surprises down the road in life.

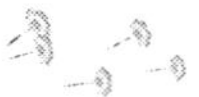

Coping mechanisms vary from person to person. But coping is not the same as living. When one of my patients was diagnosed, she remembers sobbing in the exam room, although her cancer was very treatable. I looked at her and said, "You can choose to live. We can all choose to live until we die." None of us is going to live forever. I tell my patients, "If you're looking to live forever, you're in the wrong clinic. I can't make that happen. My job is to help you not die prematurely and live until then."

I remember one day seeing another young mom who was also our pharmaceutical rep from out of town. I had not seen her since she'd had her baby, and she looked different now. Her hair was short and appeared to be a wig. I learned that she had breast cancer and was undergoing treatment using the same breast cancer drug the pharmaceutical company she worked for was manufacturing.

I was taken back when she told me her story.

"Here are your options," her surgeon had said after her diagnosis. Before he could lay out a plan, she interrupted him. "I don't mean to be rude, but there are no 'options,' plural. I have only one option," she told him. "I *must* stay alive."

While she was telling me this, there was such fire and determination in her eyes. Hers was the face of a survivor. When a patient is fighting so strongly, the whole support team from the doctors, to the nurses, to the family signs up in the same spirit. In fact, we captured her triumphant will to live in a life-size bronze sculpture outside our waiting room, her arms proudly raised in victory. A fight well fought.

There are many options in life. Sometimes we're at a crossroads and we don't know which way to choose. She chose to fight. *And she won.*

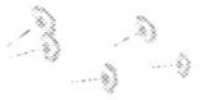

No two patients' stories are alike.

Most, however, are equally nervous (even scared) when they see me for their initial visit. I realize there is something intimidating about going to the cancer doctor for the first time. I remember a patient who seemed absolutely terrified that first day. She sat in the exam room as if she were awaiting a death sentence. However, she responded beautifully to her treatment and is now busy promoting early detection and mammography to others.

One patient used to say that she made lemonade when life handed her lemons. So many patients take their difficulty and use it for good. Some start running races. Some write books. Some dance. Some write poetry or music. Some paint on canvases, tea sets or plates. Some start support groups. Some give talks about their experience. A 90-year-old patient started painting flowers and making paper-mache out of old checks. My patients' paintings and artwork fill my workplace, and their poetry lines my walls. One of my favorite pieces of art is a woodcarving one man did for me that says, "Cancer sucks." Yes, it does.

Still, it's not a bad idea for any of us to wake up each morning and say, "Praise the Lord, I'm alive," as one of my patients does. We should all be a little more thankful and aware of each day as a gift. When one of my patients learned that her time was limited, she and her family gave themselves a gift they will never forget. They went whale watching off the West Coast, something she'd always wanted to do.

Her daughter showed me photos of her and her mother standing on the bow of the boat. My patient wore a beautiful smile and a pink raincoat with pink ribbons, her short hair tousled by the wind. They saw so many whales—more than any other boat that day. Cancer gave a mother a priceless memory with her family that none would ever forget. A year later, her family went back to repeat the trip and celebrate her life.

I was there when she talked with her family toward the end of her life. “I know you’re going to be sad when I go,” she said with a genuine smile on her face. “But I’m not.” As hard as it was to say goodbye, her family believed that the time they will spend together in the future will exceed the time they had in the past.

Live the ordinary life in an extraordinary way.

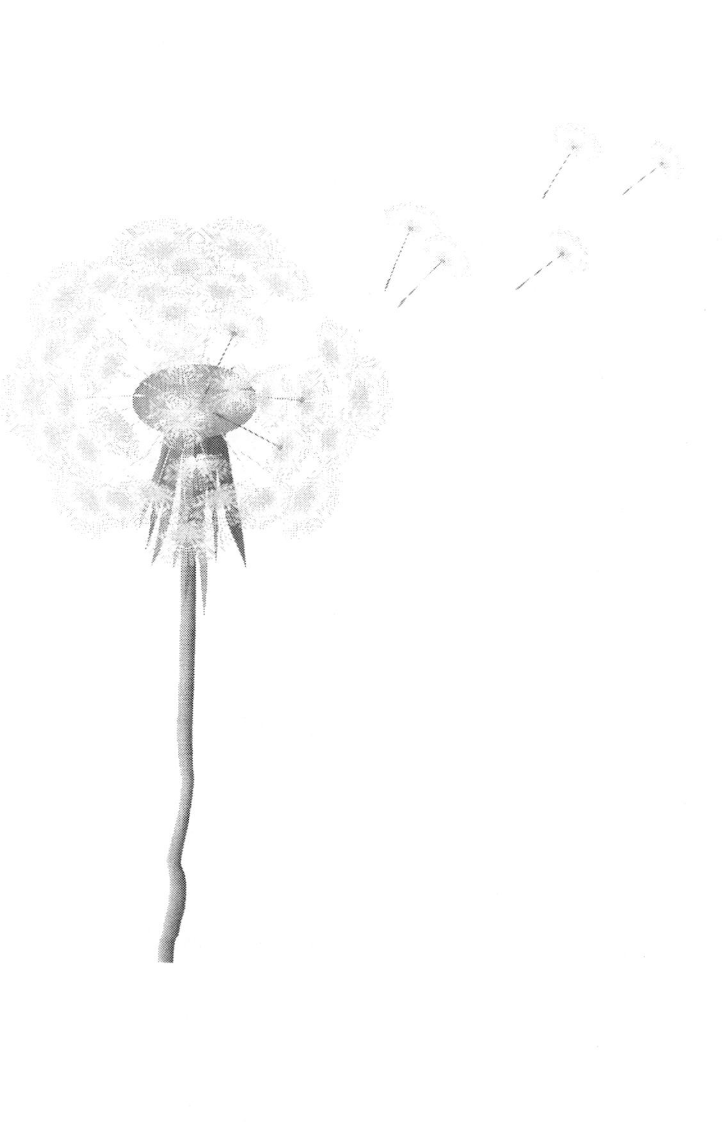

Love

I was late again.

I take my time when I'm with patients. No one likes to wait, but most patients overlook the wait when they see they receive the same personal treatment when it's their turn.

This patient had been in the crowded waiting room for a while. "Do not ever keep me waiting this long," she huffed when I finally saw her. "I have nothing in common with *those* people."

"What people?" I asked, looking around at the other cancer patients. "*You* have cancer," I reminded her. "And you have so much more in common with *these* people than you can ever imagine. You'll see."

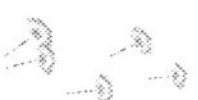

Cancer is no respecter of persons.

One of my most unforgettable patients was also learning disabled. Some of her friends called her Miss Sunshine, and she lived life to the fullest before, during and after her diagnosis. She communicated in what her family came to know as her "own language." (My friends and family say the same thing about me sometimes because of my thick accent, so I could relate!) My patient and I understood each other well nevertheless, and she knew I was there to care for her. Like so many of my patients, she was keenly aware of others the entire time she was sick. She was a frequent visitor to Disneyworld, and she often brought us mementos from her trip. She left little gifts under her parents' pillows at night—a pack of gum for her dad or a bookmark for her mom. Two weeks before she died, she ordered her parents a bouquet of flowers and thanked them for caring for her.

Her parents were so dedicated to their daughter throughout her life. When she was a child, their doctor suggested they treat her like any other child and expose her to as many experiences as possible. So, they took her everywhere with them and this unique seed—different but not defective—grew to her fullest potential under their care. She proved to me that love has its own beautiful language that everyone can understand.

In my practice, I see people from different cultures, ages and races form tight bonds on an emotional and spiritual level every day. Sadness and pain, happiness and love are timeless, universal experiences without language barriers. The only differences between us are the ones we think we have. And they're usually limited to something on the outside: what's in our wallets, even the clothes we wear. But when you're a patient in the hospital, they peel off those layers. Your wallet and clothes are removed and placed in a plastic bag. Now, wearing a hospital gown like everyone else, no outward differences remain—just bodies needing healing covered in thin, cotton gowns.

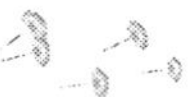

The photo on the cover of this book reminds me that life is a race that we all run together. I was working when one of my patients called me to finish the Race for the Cure with her. I came straight from the hospital to honor her request. We must take one patient at a time over the finish line. Although it's not always easy, we help each one run and finish strong one way or another.

People ask me why so many patients with cancer become passionate about helping others. Why not just focus on themselves? Some do that. But the majority of patients develop a special love for others after their experience with cancer. Many are already caregivers, and some are new to that role. But all meet on common ground where they connect, embrace and make others feel that they matter. They fight for themselves and for others in order to win.

One patient (we call her the Cake Lady) bakes two cakes every Wednesday to share with my staff and other patients. I consider what she does true artistic expression, only it's in a transient form as we devour each bite. She can make over 40 different kinds of cakes, including a rum cake that might require a designated driver. She gave up trying to name all of them long ago! The Cookie Lady comes on Mondays, making the start of another week a little easier with a tray of her oatmeal cookies. She even leaves two cookies in a brown bag for me like a mom preparing lunch for a loved one. (And it is often my early lunch!) We can't wait to admire their next piece of "art" each week.

Why have these ladies done this routine for years? To lighten the load for others. To say, "I care" in a way that every patient, young and old, can understand. Everyone wants to be heard. Everyone wants to be seen and told that they matter. When patients who have received so much kindness are finally well again, many quietly pay it forward in their own way. I realize this camaraderie is not unique to cancer survivors. Still, I'm uniquely privileged to witness it.

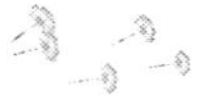

One of my patients read in my memoir that I never had a doll as a child. She came to my office one day holding a doll wearing a pink and white checkered dress and pigtails. "This is for my favorite girl," she said and placed the doll in my arms. "Lizzie," as we named her, proudly sits in a chair in my office today. Another patient occasionally left eggs and milk on my doorstep when she knew I was returning from a meeting out of town. Others leave me encouraging notes and letters on my desk.

Years ago when I was on a spiritual journey, one of my patients became more concerned about my eternal destiny, even though he was the one dying. "I know where I'm going when I die," he assured me. "But I'm not sure where my doctor is going."

The husband of another one my patients had his own way of letting me know that he cared about me as a person, not just his wife's doctor. After I finished examining his wife, he would settle back in his chair (signaling the visit was not over). Crossing his arms, he would gently ask, "And how is Dr. Vukelja doing today?" He was genuinely concerned about my family and my personal needs. Answering, "I'm fine," would not cut it. Papa, as he asked us to call him, wanted to know more. Each day he would get on his knees and pray for our entire medical team. When his wife recently found him dead at their home, he was still warm, curled down on his knees in prayer.

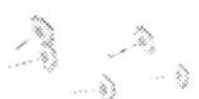

My patients remind me every day that there are no ordinary lives. I often tell my patients that they have the "extra." Cancer can become the "extra" in a life that appears "ordinary" otherwise. When patients use their cancer to enrich themselves and others, their ordinary lives are transformed forever. Only when you know their stories do you realize what effort and strength it took to get where they are. Open your eyes and see them as they really are: extraordinary. And if you've ever had the chance to love one—and be loved by one—you know exactly what I mean.

The seeds from my patients bloom all around me every day, and they are far too numerous to count. My patients have helped me through my life as much or more than I have helped them. And for that, I am grateful.

If you live each day as if it was your last,
someday you'll most certainly be right.

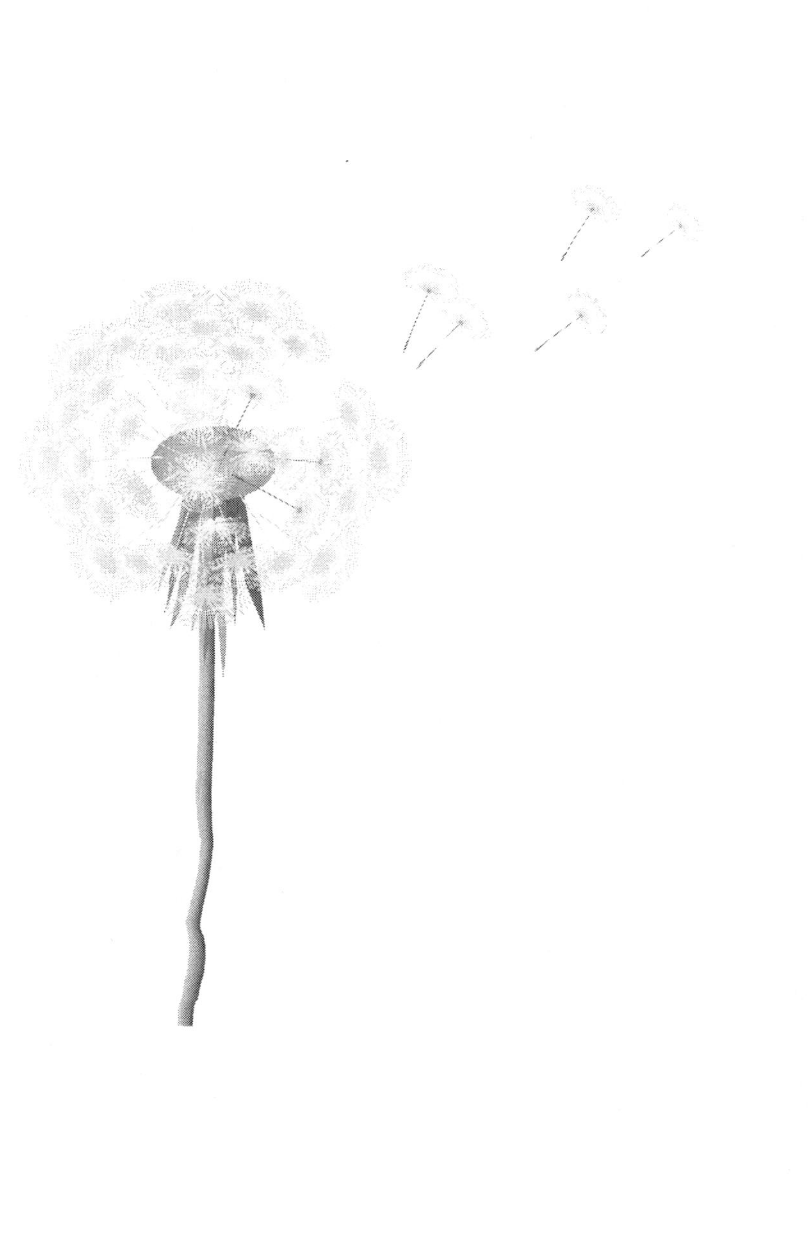

CPSIA information can be obtained at www.ICGtesting.com
Printed in the USA
LVOW011726271211

261234LV00002B/1/P

9 780578 097756